Graham Hughes

Hughes Syndrome

A Patient's Guide

Springer
London
Berlin
Heidelberg
New York
Barcelona
Hong Kong
Milan
Paris
Singapore
Tokyo

Graham Hughes
St Thomas' Hospital
Lambeth Palace Road
London SE1 7EH

British Library Cataloguing in Publication Data
Hughes, Graham, 1940–
    Hughes syndrome: a patient's guide
    I. Title
    616'.0798
    ISBN 1-85233-457-6

ISBN 1-85233-457-6 Springer-Verlag London Berlin Heidelberg

Printed in Great Britain

Typeset by Florence Production Ltd, Stoodleigh, Devon, England
Printed and bound at Latimer Trend, Plymouth, Devon, England
28/3830-543210   Printed on acid-free paper   SPIN 10797277

Foreword

The Antiphospholipid or Hughes Syndrome is not invented but is a biological aberration. In many ways, the description of a syndrome is truly a scientific effort because it is based on the accrual of data and organizing that data into something that describes an event in a large group of people. This can be a difficult task, since one has to take scientific data from a group of people with different complaints. While many such syndromes or diseases are new and have never been seen before, most have been around for years and are just now coming to light because of science. One could draw some parallels to the well-known disease lupus that was originally thought to be quite rare and of which little was known. Now the same could be said for people with the antiphospholipid syndrome the subject of this book.

The author of this book, Professor Graham Hughes and his colleagues described something in medicine for the first time. A very important disease, which affects millions of people around the world, was recognized early by Dr. Hughes. He saw something different in both the clinic and the laboratory for the first time and he was the first to call this condition the Antiphospholipid syndrome. The Antiphospholipid syndrome affects the blood and its ability to clot. The blood from patients with this illness clots too quickly and the consequences of this include strokes and heart attacks because of blood clots that go to places like the heart or brain. Fortunately, this does not happen to everyone and the disease is easily treated with blood thinners. The overall condition is caused by the same kind of antibodies or proteins directed against self; in essence a classical autoimmune disease.

No doubt, it will take many years to understand the why, how and what of this new illness, but it must be explained to the people who have it in clear fashion. My patients ask me about this condition all of the time. While an easy explanation you could say is not possible, patients deserve an explanation because they have to take the medicine, understand the precautions and the prognoses and experience the results of our therapy and our goals concerning treatment.

In this tome, Dr. Hughes considers you the patient. He has followed Louis Pasteur's aphorism that "chance favors the prepared mind". Indeed, it does since the discovery of these particular antibodies allows us to understand a complex illness and gain insight into heart disease, stroke and "hardened arteries". Now you have the opportunity to understand this unfortunate but interesting biological problem.

Read this work to understand antiphospholipid disease and the problems of autoimmunity through Dr. Hughes' masterful efforts of description. These are the diseases of our time that piece by piece provide a better understanding of our immune systems.

Robert G. Lahita M.D., Ph.D.
Professor at New York Medical College
Section Chief Rheumatology
Saint Vincent's Medical Center
New York, N.Y.

Preface

In 1983, we described a condition in which the blood has a heightened tendency to clot, and developed a blood test to diagnose this condition.

The condition, known by its rather daunting title, the Antiphospholipid Syndrome (APS) or, by many of my international colleagues as Hughes' Syndrome, is now known to be common.

The clotting can affect any vein or artery in the body, and the clinical features are diverse, varying from migraine, memory loss and strokes to leg vein thrombosis and lung clots.

In pregnancy, the clotting can affect the placenta, resulting in miscarriage.

As a physician, there are two important messages. Firstly, the condition is potentially preventable (the pregnancy success rate has increased in these patients from under 20% to over 70%.) Secondly, a simple blood test can identify it.

For me, this has been the single most rewarding discovery of my medical career – a daunting syndrome which can now be diagnosed and tamed.

This book is dedicated to my colleagues world-wide who have joined me in this research effort. It is particularly dedicated to my team in the lupus unit at St Thomas' Hospital.

January 2001

Graham Hughes
St Thomas' Hospital
London

Contents

1 Sticky Blood : the Disease Is Common

Introduction

In the early 1980's we described a group of clinical features – a syndrome – associated with "sticky blood" – a tendency for the blood to clot too easily. We found that the tendency was very clearly associated with the presence of a blood protein – a so-called "antibody" which appeared to enhance this "sticky" tendency.

This antibody, so called "antiphopsholipid antibody" (a term that will be explained later) is easily measured, and forms the basis of a standard blood test.

The antibody, if present, is a risk factor for thrombosis. While its presence does not absolutely mean that an individual will develop a clot, the chances of this occurring are certainly much greater. The presence of the antibody is particularly important during pregnancy, where the blood is slightly stickier. Here, the blood might not reach the smallest capillaries in the placenta, the developing fetus is starved of circulation and "spontaneous" abortion results.

One of the huge successes of recent medicine has been the recognition of this syndrome and the fact that treatment can prevent both the thrombotic complications and the miscarriages. For example, women with the syndrome who have had 12 or more miscarriages are now having successful pregnancies.

This brief introduction to the syndrome is dedicated both to doctors and patients.

1

For the Doctor

Do you have patients in your practice with recurrent migraine? Or with memory loss? Or with recurrent spontaneous abortions? Or with a history of deep vein thrombosis on starting the oral contraceptive therapy? Or even someone with an unexpected stroke at the age of 40?

If so, some of these patients may have a potentially treatable condition – "sticky blood" – the antiphospholipid (Hughes') syndrome – a condition which can be diagnosed by a simple and inexpensive blood antibody test.

The presence of antibodies against phospholipids is detected by two blood tests – anticardiolipin antibodies (aCL) and the confusingly named "lupus anticoagulant" (LA) test. Both of these tests are available throughout the world, and are reasonably well standardised. Perhaps more important than their role in diagnosis is the fact that they may be relevant in prevention.

To give two examples: it has been estimated that up to 1 in 5 of all strokes in the under 40 year olds are due to the syndrome.

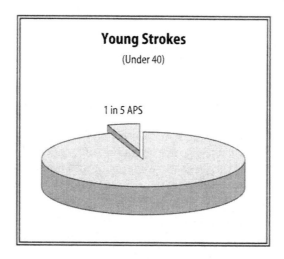

Fig. 1.1

In obstetrics, up to 25% of all women with 2 or more spontaneous miscarriages or fetal losses have Hughes' syndrome. Both are examples where a blood test and preventative (prophylactic) treatment, often with as simple an agent as junior aspirin, could have huge clinical and economic implications.

There are a number of known causes of the "sticky blood" clotting tendency, but the antiphospholipid syndrome (APS) is uniquely important in its frequency and in its potential for both venous and arterial thrombosis.

It is a sure bet that the syndrome is seen in every branch of medicine, from psychiatry to neurology, from obstetrics to general practice.

This is not a rare syndrome, it is common, and is potentially treatable.

For the Patient

The range of symptoms which the patient with Hughes' syndrome can develop is daunting.

Little wonder, therefore, that many patients go from doctor to doctor before the diagnosis is made.

In some, the diagnosis is immediate and dramatic – the leg vein thrombosis on the oral contraceptive "pill", for example, or the sudden headache and speech disturbance suggestive of an early stroke.

In others, it can be difficult – especially where more "subtle" brain clotting occurs – the memory loss (and fear of "Alzheimers"), the headaches, the balance disturbance, the periods of "petit mal" or absences. In others, the problems seem to relate mostly to pregnancy – or pregnancy failure, with recurrent pregnancy loss, and even, in some women, with infertility.

The basis of the syndrome is a tendency of the blood to clot spontaneously. Nature normally protects the body from "inappropriate" clotting. However, in Hughes' syndrome, circulating proteins called antibodies appear to make the blood far more "sticky" and liable to clot. In an analogy with the car engine, if the petrol or gas mixture is too rich, the engine cokes up, stutters, and ceases to function properly.

The disease is treatable: clearly treatment demands one or other form of blood-thinning agents.

Obviously, in a disease which affects the blood and the blood vessels, any organ or the body may be affected. The results (and therefore the symptoms) can vary enormously. In the brain, for example, the effects can range from the extreme – a stroke, to the more subtle, for example, early memory loss.

3

Perhaps one of the biggest mysteries of the syndrome is what triggers the thrombosis. Indeed, an important question is why so many individuals carrying the antibodies *don't* appear to thrombose. Maybe some or many "asymptomatic" carriers will develop thrombosis in time – but as yet the syndrome is still less than 20 years old!

2 Main Clinical Features

There are two main clinical features – clotting (thrombosis) and, in women, recurrent miscarriage. In the blood, the defining test is the presence of antiphospholipid antibodies (aPL) (see Chapter 15).

There are enormous variations in presentation and in severity of Hughes' Syndrome, most, though not all, being explained on a basis of blood clotting. It is important to recognise that in this syndrome, as distinct from other (usually less common) clotting disorders, the thrombosis may happen both in the veins and in the arteries – the latter with much more severe consequences. The major features of the syndrome are listed in table 2.1.

What Are the Signs?

For obvious reasons, the majority of cases currently seen by us have been diagnosed either because they have had a sudden clot, e.g., a leg thrombosis ("DVT") or recurrent clots, or else because they have been

Table 2.1. Hughes' Syndrome – major clinical features

1. Vein thrombosis	• Deep vein thrombosis (DVT) e.g. arm or leg.
	• Thrombosis in internal organs, e.g. kidney, liver, lung, brain, eye
	• Thrombosis of skin vessels – skin ulcers "Livedo" (blotchiness)
2. Artery thrombosis	• Brain – headaches, weakness, slurred speech ("transient ischaemic attacks" – "TIA's"), strokes, seizures, memory loss
	• Limb – pain, circulation problems, other organs – heart, kidney, adrenal
3. Pregnancy loss	• Early in pregnancy (miscarriage) or late ("fetal death")
	• Recurrent very early miscarriage may give rise to diagnosis of infertility
4. Low platelet count	• Bruising (5–20%)

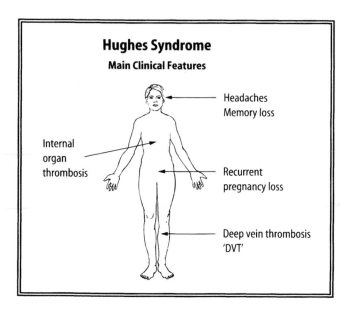

Fig. 2.1

referred by an obstetrician who has made the diagnosis by aPL testing in a woman who has had a number of miscarriages.

In some, the history may be sudden, with the development of features suggestive of an early stroke or "transient ischaemic attack".

In others, the history may be longer, with, for example, headaches, or memory loss going back over a number of years.

The disease affects all age groups, from infancy (see later) to old age. However, the majority of patients are aged between 15 and 50. Females seem to outnumber males, though not to any great extent. These observations on age and sex may be flawed in that "referral patterns" may influence the figures. For example, because of the known association with pregnancy loss, there may well be a selection bias from pregnancy clinics.

What Triggers the Thrombosis?

There are well known factors contributing to thrombosis in general : these include smoking, immobility (e.g. long flights), dehydration, and the contraceptive pill.

6

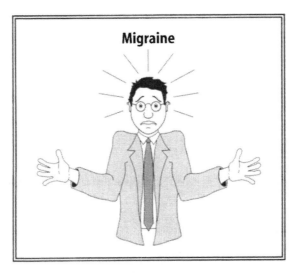

Fig. 2.2

Pregnancy itself causes a slight increase in blood stickiness and it may be that this in itself contributes to the proclivity of syndrome to present during pregnancy. It has been mentioned there is a slight genetic tendency to the disease, and there may be a family history of clots, of miscarriage, or of other "auto-immune" diseases such as lupus and thyroid problems.

Occasionally, and of great interest to research workers, the thrombosis seems to happen during an infection such as a sore throat.

Despite these obvious triggers, in the vast majority of patients, the thrombosis seems to happen "out of the blue". In some of these patients the past history – recurrent migraine, recurrent miscarriages, for example – suggest that the syndrome had been present, if undiagnosed, for years.

Positive Blood Tests

This brings us to one of the most difficult problems – one that we are facing with increased frequency. What of the "asymptomatic" individual found to have aPL on routine blood screening.

It is my own belief that the present of aPL is an *important* risk factor for thrombosis.. It may well be that one day aPL screening will become not

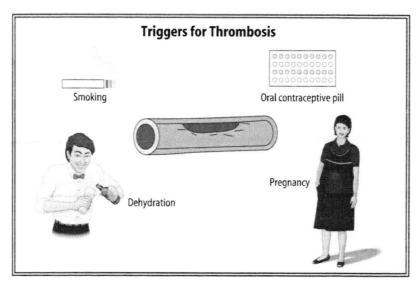

Fig. 2.3

only part of the testing of women with two or more miscarriages or fetal losses, or those with recurrent thrombosis or "early" strokes, but more widespread. A test that costs a few dollars, which could potentially prevent strokes, pregnancy tragedies and thrombosis, could arguably be as important a screening test as cholesterol screening is today.

3 Clotting in Veins

The commonest veins to be affected are those in the leg – commonly referred to as "deep vein thrombosis" or DVT However, "internal" veins may be involved in delicate organs such as the kidney, eye or brain.

An interesting observation has been made that, when a further or "recurrent" thrombosis occurs, it often follows a similar pattern, i.e., those with vein thrombosis are more prone to further vein thrombosis, while artery clots may be followed by further arterial clots. Although not *absolutely* correct, this clinical generalisation does have potentially important implications, especially when it comes to making long term treatment decisions about the length and intensity of anti-clotting treatment regimes.

Limb Thrombosis

The "classical" presentation of a "DVT" in the leg is of sudden calf pain and swelling. Pointing the foot upwards causes pain in the calf ("Homan's sign").

The whole leg may become swollen and tight. Although the diagnosis may be clinically obvious, it usually needs to be clinically confirmed by investigations such as ultrasound.

Traditionally, DVT's are a recognised complication of surgery, especially gynaecological or pelvic surgery (where there may be more obstruction of blood flow from the leg), and of prolonged immobility, especially long flights.

CASE REPORT
A 48 year old woman developed pain and swelling in the right leg on a flight from Singapore to London. She was found to have a deep vein thrombosis. She was a non-smoker and had not drunk alcohol on the

plane. Two years later, she developed a further "spontaneous" leg vein thrombosis. Investigations showed positive aPL tests and she has subsequently remained symptom free on "junior" aspirin 75mgs daily.

One well known predisposing factor in the development of thrombosis is the oral contraceptive pill. It may be that the APS proves to be an important deterring factor in the known link between the pill and thrombosis.

CASE REPORT

A 17 year old girl was started on the oral contraceptive pill. There were no known predisposing risk factors to thrombosis with one possible exception – a history of previous occasional migraine attacks, present since the age of 13.

Within 2 weeks of starting the pill she collapsed. She was found to have major thrombosis in the leg veins with spread of the clot to the pelvic veins and the lungs. She survived following a prolonged period of intensive care. She has high levels of aPL and has since been treated successfully with Warfarin (Coumadin). Three years later aPL levels remain high and Warfarin treatment continues. She is now married and considering pregnancy.

The issues raised by this case concern not only treatment (see chapter 13) but also the wider and important issue of prevention (should migraine sufferers be tested for aPL? – yes, in my opinion).

Thrombosis in the Arm   While less common, this can be equally dramatic. Often occurring at night (it was once suggested that a tight pyjama sleeve might precipitate it), the presentation is with a painful, swollen arm, often with prominent looking veins on the arms and upper chest.

Lung   The major concern in DVT patients is the risk of a spread to the lung. Although a clot in the leg or pelvic veins may seem to be stable, this is often not the case and a segment of clot can "break off" and travel up to the lung. The picture of a so-called "pulmonary embolus" is of sudden chest pain – often in one or other side of the chest, especially on deep inspiration.

Pulmonary embolus can be extremely serious – even fatal – and is a major medical emergency. Other clinical features are of acute shortness of breath, light headedness, cough, sometimes with bloody sputum, and collapse.

The clinical diagnosis is usually confirmed if possible with scanning ("VQ scan") which shows impaired blood supply in the affected area of the lung. Urgent anti-clotting treatment is vital and in rare cases, emergency surgical removal of the clot can be life-saving.

Fortunately, extreme and fatal cases of pulmonary embolism complicate only a minority of DVT's. At the other extreme, subtle and recurrent smaller pulmonary clots can be undiagnosed.

CASE REPORT
A 44 year old man developed increasing shortness of breath over a 2 year period. He was a non-smoker and had little in the way of a cough. After extensive investigations, lung scanning revealed numerous areas of lung clotting ("pulmonary infarction"). He was found to have high titres of aPL but had given no past history of significance.

One rare, but extremely important and serious complication in some patients with aPL is so-called "**pulmonary hypertension**". In this condition, the patient, who complains of gradually worsening shortness of breath on exertion, is found to have an increased (pathologically high) pressure in the lung arteries. In most patients, the cause of this serious condition is unknown. However, in our description of the syndrome in 1983, we reported pulmonary hypertension as an association of aPL. Presumably the raised pressure results from a gradual process of clotting and narrowing of the lung vessels.

Some patients with pulmonary hypertension are known to have aPL and in others there is a past history of clots, or of migraine or of previous repeated miscarriages. There is now a collaborative European study group looking at this disease to see whether any cases could, in future, be prevented.

Liver   The liver is an important organ in the metabolism of food and drugs. Thrombosis of liver veins is now well recognised in patients with APS. Most commonly, the first indication comes with routine blood tests, where "liver function tests" are found to be abnormal.

For many years, a rather mysterious condition of thrombosis of the main "hepatic portal vein" was known as the Budd-Chiari syndrome. In many cases the cause was unknown.

CASE REPORT
A 21 year old female Indian student with a long history of discoid lupus (an autoimmune skin condition) was admitted to hospital with anaemia

and blood loss from the stomach and oesophagus veins. She was found to have abnormal liver function tests and thrombosis of the main vein to the liver.

(This patient, described in our original series of patients in 1983, is alive and well 17 years later, on long-term anticoagulant treatment.)

For doctors dealing with Hughes' syndrome, abnormal liver function tests should point towards a clotting problem in the liver blood supply.

Kidney Renal vein thrombosis is a well recognised acute medical problem. Again, the majority of cases have no known cause, but APS is now recognised as an important contributor in some cases.

The clinical picture is often dramatic – there is loin pain (the kidney becomes swollen) and the urine contains increasing amounts of leaked protein.

Sometimes, so much protein is lost that the body's metabolism is upset, leading to marked ankle swelling and fluid retention. The recognition of this rare complication of APS is vital as urgent treatment can save the kidney from permanent damage.

CASE REPORT
A 34 year old patient, at 35 weeks of pregnancy, developed severe weight gain, leg swelling and fluid retention. She was found to have high levels of protein in the urine. Investigations showed that she had thrombosis in the veins from both kidneys ("renal vein thrombosis"). The baby was delivered successfully but the patient went on to develop severe kidney problems. She was anticardiolipin positive on blood testing.

Eye Both the veins and, more seriously, the arteries of the eye can develop thrombosis. Clotting in these vessels lead to visual symptoms such as flickering vision, temporary visual loss, and loss of parts of the visual field. Recognition of the symptoms, their relationship to "sticky blood" and, of course, prompt treatment with anticoagulants can save the sight.

Brain Although the major worry of Hughes' syndrome is of arterial thrombosis (strokes), the veins in and around the brain can also be prone to thrombosis. One well-described area has been thrombosis of the saggital sinus (the main vein over the top of the brain), leading to a damming back of fluid in the brain – a condition known as "benign intracranial hypertension" ("benign" because another, different cause of the condition is brain tumour).

CASE REPORT

A 22 year old male student, whilst on a climbing expedition high in the Andes, collapsed, became unconscious, and only recovered after being given emergency treatment, and hospital management at lower altitude. Subsequent investigations showed that he had developed a saggital sinus thrombosis and was aPL positive.

This case is interesting in possibly supporting the "two hit" hypothesis in APS – the underlying problem ("sticky blood") and the precipitating factor – in this case possibly high altitude and its associated metabolic changes.

While vein thrombosis can and does occasionally affect the brain, the main concern with this organ, and, indeed, for all patients with Hughes' syndrome, is the risk of strokes. It is this threat which makes diagnosis and screening for APS so important, and decisions concerning duration and intensity of treatment so critical.

In a perverse way, the brain can be viewed as a simple organ. If angered or insulted, it is capable of reacting in fairly limited, well defined ways.

Just as the car engine starved of fuel either stutters or stops, so the brain, if given limited blood (and hence oxygen) supply, complains in ways well

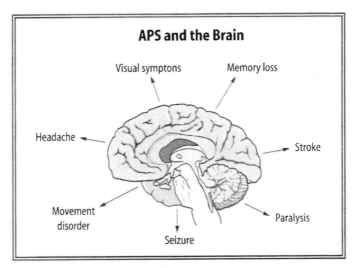

Fig. 3.1

13

recognised by the neurologist. The most dramatic and serious, of course, is a stroke, with weakness down one side of the body and possibly with effects on speech. More localised ischaemia (poor circulation) can lead to a wide variety of features including seizures, migraine, visual disturbance, spinal cord problems.

Some patients present with less "dramatic" symptoms – such as memory loss, loss of sensation (sometimes leading to a mistaken diagnosis of "multiple sclerosis", movement disorders (including chorea – "St Vitus Dance").

Although the threat of the development of a stroke is the biggest fear, one wonders how many individuals with more subtle forms of brain involvement are either being misdiagnosed, or not being diagnosed at all.

4 Stroke

Throughout the world, stroke is not only a major personal disaster, but an economic and social problem of huge proportions. In the UK, for example, it has been estimated that stroke is number one in terms of national medical expenditure, accounting for over 10% of the annual National Health Service budget.

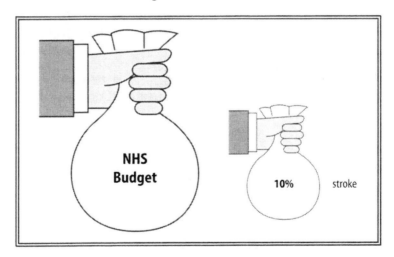

Fig. 4.1

There are some well known and preventable causes of stroke, such as high blood pressure. Having said this, in the majority of cases, the cause is unknown. Thus, the finding of a new, and potentially preventable cause – "sticky blood" – the antiphospholipid syndrome (APS) – is reason for celebration – and for further medical research.

Some years ago we carried out a study in Barcelona with Dr Xavier Montalban and his neurology colleagues there. When we looked at all stroke patients coming to the hospital, whatever their age, we found the APS in 7%. A subsequent study from Dr Nencini and colleagues in Rome, looked at "young" strokes, i.e., under the age of 45. Here the percentage associated with aPL rose dramatically to 16%. Thus, in any "unexpected" stroke in an individual aged, say, 40 or younger, one might expect up to 1 in 5 to have the APS.

This has huge implications in management. In many medical circles, stroke is often traditionally thought of as being more commonly due to bleeding rather than clotting. The finding of aPL might help in the decision to anticoagulate. In many patients, there are "transient" or warning strokes – presumably following similar clotting or sluggish brain circulation, but without leading to permanent damage.

CASE REPORT
A 26 year old previously fit building labourer became unwell at a railway station whilst going to a sports fixture with friends. He suffered a headache and, according to his friends, started "speaking gibberish". The speech disturbance lasted approximately 15 minutes. On admission to hospital, he had slight weakness on one side of the face. His brain scan was normal and he made a full recovery. He remembered suffering a similar but less severe episode some 3 months previously. He was found to be aPL positive and was subsequently treated with Warfarin (Coumadin).

Scanning techniques have helped in diagnosis. The magnetic resonance imaging (MRI) scan is the most widely used. Areas of brain damage due to a lack of oxygen show up as white areas. Varying in size from the pinprick to larger prominent areas. In some patients, the MRI resembles the sky at night.

This is not the place for discussion of the merits of different forms of scan. Suffice it to say that improvements in scanning techniques are now having an impact on our ability to detect smaller lesions.

One of the most consistent – and most remarkable clinical observations is the improvement seen in many patients when appropriate anticoagulation treatment is started. In Chapter 13 I will be returning to this theme. There are many, many patients who know *precisely* when their medical control is correct – and when it is not correct.

CASE REPORT
An internationally famous author aged 46 had previously been diagnosed as having Hughes' syndrome, having had a variety of symptoms,

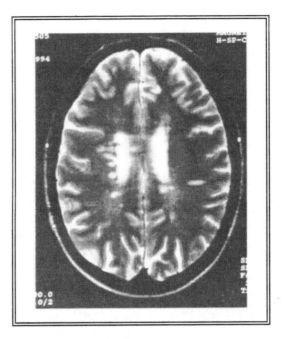

Fig. 4.2

including visual disturbance, speech disturbance ("talking rubbish") and the bizarre symptom of writing inappropriate words or even whole sentences in her text. She was successfully treated with Warfarin

The anti-clotting control "INR" (see treatment chapter) was generally good, but whenever the INR fell below 3.2 (and precisely 3.2), the patient again developed headaches, speech disturbance and writing "gobbledygook".

It is not difficult to imagine that there are literally thousands of individuals with similar, or perhaps more subtle manifestations of "sludging" of the brain circulation. So many of my patients have expressed the worry that they might be suffering from Alzheimer's disease.

5 Memory Loss and "Alzheimers"

Here we come to the single most important feature of the syndrome – at least in my view. Recurrent pregnancy loss and strokes are both major medical problems where the importance of aPL testing is becoming recognised. Not so in the case of memory loss. At the time of writing, there are few "cognitive" studies of Hughes' syndrome patients – either before or after treatment.

And yet it is here that many of the most dramatic stories are heard. Asking the patient about memory loss sometimes opens the floodgates – "I'm so glad you asked, I hadn't wanted to mention it". "I'm the joke of the family and now have to write everything down". "I thought I was developing Alzheimer's disease".

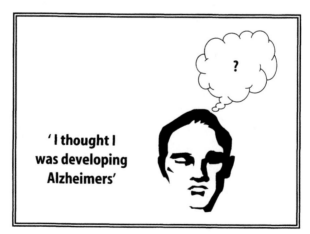

Fig. 5.1

Obviously a clot can cause any variety of nervous system features, depending on the size, the frequency, and, critically, on the site of the thrombosis.

CASE REPORT

A 40 year old woman, the champion of her country village darts team, suddenly became unable to "hit the 20" – she couldn't recognise its number or position. She was found to have APS and, on brain scan (MRI) had one small area of clot.

CASE REPORT

A 38 year old South African female musician started to become forgetful and made mistakes on the keyboard. Within a year she had to give up her job with a travelling band. She had a past history of miscarriages and of migraine and developed slurred speech and a "drunken" gait on walking. She was found to have widespread areas of brain ischaemia (brain damage due to impaired circulation) and blood tests revealed high titres of aPL. She has been started on life-long anticoagulation with Warfarin (Coumadin).

I am sure that one day the syndrome will become widely recognised by psychologists and psychiatrists as an important differential diagnosis in some individuals with "neuro-psychiatric" or "cognitive" disorders. My last 2 case reports in this section highlight some of the diagnostic difficulties at either end of the age spectrum.

CASE REPORT

A 4 year old boy was referred from Italy for advice regarding management. He had developed a marked personality disorder, with aggressive behaviour, poor memory and with one seizure. Investigations revealed multiple lesions, especially in the frontal (front) cortex area of the brain. He was aPL positive. He has been started on Warfarin – probably for life.

CASE REPORT

A highly successful 52 year old school teacher at one of London's leading schools, started to complain of memory loss, fatigue and a lack of drive and energy. There were occasional headaches. She was investigated but no diagnosis was made. A course of anti-depressants was unhelpful. She was unable to continue in her job. Three years later, she developed a stroke, thought initially to be due to a brain haemorrhage, but subsequently thought to be due to a blood clot. It was soon after this that she was found to have positive aPL. After discussion, it was decided to start Warfarin. The result was dramatic. There was a disappearance of the mental sluggishness and fatigue, and a return to a reasonably normal life. Like many other patients, she "knows" precisely when the anticoagulant control ("INR") has slipped – the headaches and "foggy brain" return.

These short case reports underline, I believe, the importance of diagnosis and correct management of the syndrome. The brain features, whilst often subtle enough to go undiagnosed, are devastating for the patient who suffers them.

6 Headaches, Migraine and Fits

Headaches and Migraine

The case reports in the previous chapters point to the importance of headaches as a feature of APS. In many cases, the headaches are accompanied by the flashing lights, nausea and vomiting of a true migraine. In many more, they vary in character.

Interestingly, many patients give "past histories" of migraine or severe headaches in their teens. To date, few studies have been carried out on large groups of migraine sufferers. My prediction is that APS will become an important recognised cause of migraine: even more important when one considers the link (unusual, but definite) between migraine and stroke, and between migraine and adverse reactions to the oral contraceptive pill.

It is clinically interesting to have observed that a number of our APS patients find a marked improvement in the severity and frequency of the headaches when junior aspirin treatment is started. Even more tantalising to me is the observation that in some of my APS patients with intractable migraine, there is complete resolution when anticoagulation is started.

Recently, we have, in some patients, embarked on a policy of short clinical "trial" of anticoagulation for 2 weeks, to assess response. Daily self-administration of heparin (in our study, low molecular weight delteparin ("Fragmin") 10,000 units daily for 2 weeks) is proving a useful guide to response – in some patients the headaches disappearing completely.

21

Fits and Seizures

The brain's list of responses to insult is limited. One of the most dramatic is with fits or seizures. Fortunately, a feature in only the minority of patients with Hughes' syndrome, it is nevertheless important to recognise the association. All types of fits have been described, including petit mal ("absences"), temporal lobe epilepsy (with its unusual characteristics such as "déjà vu") and grand mal (seizures).

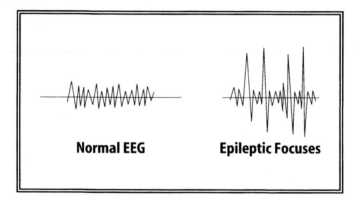

Normal EEG   **Epileptic Focuses**

Fig. 6.1

In most cases the fits are limited to a first or major event, and recurrent fits are uncommon. However, the following case report throws up some interesting observations.

CASE REPORT

A 42 year old wife of an American diplomat had a past history of lupus (see Chapter 12), now well controlled on a small dose of steroids (5mgs prednisolone daily). Her major problem, and one with a major impact on her busy life, was recurrent seizures – both petit mal and grand mal, for which she had received a variety of combinations of anti-epileptic treatment. On examination, the only abnormality was a blotchy skin appearance known as livedo. Blood tests showed the lupus to be inactive, but she had extremely high levels of antiphospholipid antibodies. During her stay in London she developed a DVT of the leg and routine anticoagulation with Warfarin (Coumadin) was started. An immediate, and unexpected bonus, was a marked reduction and severity of the seizures – requiring far less aggressive anti-epileptic treatment.

It is difficult to explain the improvement following anticoagulation when the problem has been long-standing. Nevertheless, that's what happened. In fact, it is an observation which has been made in another fairly long-standing problem – chorea.

Movement Disorders

Chorea (St Vitus' Dance) is a peculiar repetitive abnormal movement, affecting particularly the limbs. The symptoms vary between sudden "jerking" movements, especially in the arms, to more sinuous "Thai dancing" complex movements.

In former times, chorea was a recognised complication of rheumatic fever (a streptococcus infection) but, in Western countries at least, rheumatic fever is now rare. Despite this, some patients with Hughes' syndrome or with lupus are wrongly diagnosed as having rheumatic fever – perhaps not too surprisingly as both conditions can give rise to chorea, heart murmurs and aches and pains.

In most patients with APS, the chorea is a transient feature. In others, it is more persistent. Thus, it is rather surprising that occasional cases improve when anticoagulation is started. I know of 4 such cases, 2 under our care here at St Thomas', and one each under the care of Dr Angela Tincani in Italy and Dr Ron Derksen in Holland.

7 The Spinal Cord and "Multiple Sclerosis"

Spinal Cord Problems

Our early work on antiphospholipid antibodies was on the spinal cord disease "Jamaican neuropathy". So, in a way, it came as no surprise when we saw some APS patients with spinal cord lesions. Perhaps next to stroke, this is the most feared complication of APS. Damage to this region can paralyse the lower limbs as well as the bladder. Spinal cord disease has long been a feature of lupus, and some have suggested that the presence of aPL and thrombosis is the link in many of these cases. Fortunately, this is a rare problem, and there is still insufficient data to say whether anticoagulation (in addition to the more conventional steroid treatment) is the treatment of choice.

Anecdotally, this treatment *did* work – dramatically – in one of our patients.

CASE REPORT
A 36 year old housewife known to have mild lupus, developed progressive paralysis of the lower limbs. She was confined to a wheelchair and the spasms in the legs became so severe that on more than one occasion she was thrown from the chair. Investigations in a neuro-surgical unit revealed an unusual vascular malformation (and "arterio-venous" malformation) in the spinal cord. The neurologists' opinion was that the symptoms seemed far too severe for the degree of malformation seen. Her blood contained high titres of aPL. Perhaps here were 2 contributing factors – "sticky blood" and an abnormal blood pathway for it to flow through. Logic suggested a trial of anticoagulants and we started Warfarin. The result has been gratifying. The patient now lives, works, walks (and dances) normally.

The Eye

As has been mentioned, a cut off of blood supply to the eye can have a variety of effects. Perhaps the most common is a loss of part of the field of vision, either in one or both eyes. The nervous supply to and from the eyes is well documented, and by studying the area of visual loss on a standard screen an assessment can be made of the approximate site of the lesion.

As in other fields of medicine the recognition of APS is making inroads into the assessment and treatment of patients with sudden visual loss.

Balance

Some APS patients complain that their balance is affected. In a small number, intense vertigo suggestive of middle ear disease has been a prominent and distressing feature.

It is possible that in such cases, thrombosis affecting the blood supply to the middle ear is the cause. A number of studies are underway to investigate middle ear involvement in Hughes' syndrome.

Multiple Sclerosis

Mention the brain, the eye, the spinal cord and the possibility of a diagnosis of multiple sclerosis is raised. Thus, it is not surprising that a number of patients are wrongly diagnosed as "MS".

CASE REPORT
A 23 year old neurophysiology student developed headaches, occasional movement disorders, slight difficulty with gait and visual disturbance. Brain scanning (MRI) showed two small lesions, and a diagnosis of "possible MS" was made. The student's future was uncertain. She also went on to develop a low platelet count in the blood, a possible thrombosis in the leg and increasing migraines. She was found to be aPL positive, and the diagnosis was changed to Hughes' syndrome. Following the leg DVT, she was anticoagulated and has remained well since. There have been no new neurological features in 5 years' follow-up.

As the similarities between "MS" and APS can be so great, it is little wonder that the two can be confused. In the space of 3 months, Dr Maria Cuadrado, working in our unit, identified 27 such patients.

This study was of particular interest to us. When we look back at those cases of MS who were subsequently found to have Hughes' Syndrome, treatment with anticoagulants resulted in almost complete arrest of the illness.

The implications hardly need rehearsing – MS is a largely untreatable disease. APS on the other hand is both detectable *and* potentially treatable. The two diseases are altogether different. But it seems a sure bet that many more APS patients labouring under the incorrect "MS" diagnosis will be identified. Watch this space!

8 The Heart and Arteries

Heart Valves

There are 2 areas of the heart which can be affected – the heart valves, and the heart's own coronary arteries.

One of the stranger aspects of the APS in sicker, usually untreated patients is the development of heart valve lesions. In extreme cases, lumps of thrombosis (clot) develop on the valves, especially the mitral and aortic valves.

These can impair normal blood flow, and, more seriously, can dislodge and fly off to affect other organs.

This valve involvement is one of the many features which separates APS from other clotting disorders. Milder cases usually go undetected, but are sometimes picked up as a heart murmur on stethoscope examination of the chest. The diagnosis is more precisely confirmed by echo-cardiography – a painless and quick chest examination.

Echo-cardiography has been part of the routine screen in our APS clinic, following the studies of my colleague Dr Munther Khamashta, one of the first to draw attention to the frequency of valve disease in Hughes' syndrome.

The majority of patients with mild disease require little therapy. Rarely, however, the development of valve thrombosis and damage can be dramatic.

CASE REPORT
A 19 year old student was taken ill on a working summer vacation in Scandinavia. Over the course of 2 weeks, she became increasingly unwell, tired and short of breath. She rapidly became more short of breath and finally collapsed. In hospital she was found to have an abnormal mitral valve. She underwent heart surgery, where a clot the

size of a table-tennis ball was found on the valve, and removed. She was subsequently found to be aPL positive.

Heart Attack

As with arteries elsewhere in the body, coronary thrombosis ("heart attack") can occur in Hughes' syndrome.

Clinically, there is an impression that significant coronary thrombosis is perhaps less frequent than clotting episodes in the brain. Nevertheless, the discovery of the APS has important lessons in the field of cardiology, and of cardiac surgery.

It may well be that APS individuals with heart attack require more aggressive and precise anticoagulation than those without. To give an example, one study from Sydney showed that APS patients undergoing coronary bypass procedure had a higher risk of re-thrombosis post-operatively than those without.

Other Arteries

The fact that Hughes' syndrome patients can and do develop *arterial* as well as vein thrombosis, is of immense clinical importance. Any artery can be affected including the largest arteries such as the carotid (neck), aorta, arm and leg arteries. Again, the onset can be dramatic, as in the case of one of our patients first seen in the late 1970's.

CASE REPORT
An 18 year old boy, previously fit, and having recently won admission to university, complained of severe left calf pain. He rapidly developed painful discoloration of the foot and subsequently required amputation of the toes. Subsequent investigation revealed very high levels of aPL. The was treated with anticoagulants and has remained well (on anti-coagulants) for the past 2 decades. For the whole of this period of observation, his aPL levels have remained high.

Perhaps the most common – certainly the most well known symptoms of peripheral artery disease is so-called "intermittent claudication". The patient develops pain in the calf on walking – the pain goes away if he or she rests, but returns on further walking.

Modern tests of blood flow including the "Doppler" have made assessment of artery blood flow much more precise.

Finally, one feature of peripheral arterial disease which is recognised in other vascular diseases, but not, to my knowledge, yet described in Hughes' syndrome, is *impotence*.

CASE REPORT

A 60 year old male was referred to our APS clinic with previous thrombosis, skin "livedo", and worsening calf pains on walking. Until very recently he had received no long term treatment. Despite his many problems, the one development which concerned him most was of impotence – a problem which only come to light late on during the consultation. Significantly, this symptom was helped by the introduction of the drug sildenafil ("Viagra"). Impotence can be a problem in any disease which affects the circulation.

Artery disease is one of the major afflictions of Western society. Diet, cholesterol, smoking, life-style and genetics have all come under scrutiny. Now we have a new clue – a link between clotting or sludging of blood and the "furring up" of arteries. More important, it is a cause that can be dealt with.

9 Internal Organs

The Kidneys

As well as the heart and the brain, it is obvious that no organ in the body is immune from the risk of thrombosis due to "sticky blood".

Thrombosis of the kidney vein has already been discussed. Thrombosis of the kidney artery gives rise to a wholly different picture – that of raised blood pressure.

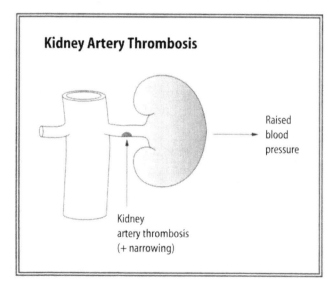

Kidney Artery Thrombosis

Raised blood pressure

Kidney artery thrombosis (+ narrowing)

Fig. 9.1

It has been known for many decades that narrowing (or damage) of the renal artery resulted in raised blood pressure. We have seen a number of patients in our APS clinic who have had raised blood pressure, and, on investigation, been found to have "renal artery stenosis" (narrowed main blood supply to the kidney). Again, this finding could have wider implications, especially in the field of kidney medicine – nephrology – where the condition of "renal artery stenosis" is well recognised, but, in most cases without any idea of the cause. If APS causes kidney artery narrowing by gradually clotting or silting up the artery, then appropriate anticoagulant treatment might seem the logical way forward in those patients found to have positive aPL and "sticky blood".

Liver and Gut

Thrombosis of the liver veins has been discussed. Thrombosis of *arteries*, though less common, is also seen occasionally.

The blood supply to the gut has also been found compromised in a small number of patients. It is a condition which is difficult to diagnose, but sometimes the symptoms are very suggestive – stomach pain coming on some time after a meal.

CASE REPORT
A 62 year old woman complained of increasingly severe stomach pains over a 2 year period. Barium meal and endoscopic examination of the esophagus, stomach and duodenum showed no abnormality. Over time it became clear that the pain followed a meal by a clear interval of about 1 hour – a symptom sometimes suggestive of "ischaemia" (i.e., not enough blood supply for the work of digestion). An x-ray investigation of the blood vessels (angiogram) showed an area of narrowing of a critical part of the major bowel artery. She was also noted clinically to have "livedo" of the skin and found to be aPL positive. She was treated surgically to remove the obstruction in the artery, and has since been on anticoagulants. The abdominal pain has gone.

Adrenal Glands

So far the syndrome has touched on the fields of neurology, cardiology, obstetrics, psychiatry and gastro-enterology. The endocrine specialist is not left out – in APS, there may be clotting involving endocrine glands such as the pituitary and the adrenals.

31

The adrenal glands are important in maintaining a variety of means of protection against stress. When the adrenal glands "fail", the common symptoms are of lethargy, fluid problems, and finally, coma.

In 1987 a young man taught us that the adrenals could be involved – dramatically – in the APS.

CASE REPORT

A 24 year old male student was referred for advice regarding treatment. He had been diagnosed in Indonesia with APS, having suffered recurrent thrombosis, with positive aPL tests in Jakarta. Almost immediately on arrival in London, he developed a further thrombosis and was admitted to hospital. He was ill and drowsy and within 24 hours became unconscious.

The diagnosis was made by a very bright junior doctor on our team who suggested that the loss of consciousness was due to chemical (electrolyte) imbalance, possibly due to failure of the adrenal gland. The patient was treated successfully and subsequent investigation showed that both adrenal glands had failed, almost certainly due to clotting in the adrenal arteries.

This particular, dramatic, case raised a lot of interest in medical circles. Dr Ron Asherson, a senior clinical fellow who joined my unit, collected, in seemingly no time at all, some 40 similar cases following our ward round discussions of this case. It so happened that a meeting on Addison's disease was being held at Guy's Hospital in London to commemorate the 200th anniversary of the birth of Thomas Addison (a Guy's doctor).

The causes of Addison's disease are varied (in the old days, tuberculosis was a major cause), but as usual, the commonest cause is "unknown". We were invited as a "late entry" to present our data on the APS as a cause (possibly an important cause) of Addison's disease.

The Skin

One of the strangest (and most striking) clinical signs of Hughes' syndrome is "livedo".

This is a blotchy appearance of the veins of the skin – hard to describe, but, once seen, never forgotten. It is a lacy, prominent "map of the world" type picture of blood vessels in the skin, most commonly seen on the knees but also seen elsewhere, for example, on the back of the wrist (under the wrist watch) and on the thighs and arms. It resembles the normal blotchiness seen in many "cold-blooded" individuals in winter – but in APS, tends to be more persistent. It is not a *specific* sign of APS, but, taken together with other pointers to the disease, it is an *important* physical sign.

One of the unusual but very distressing clinical problems in APS is skin ulceration.

Most commonly, this occurs on the legs, especially around the shins and ankles. The ulcers are due to thrombosis, and it may be difficult to make the link between leg ulcers and a clotting problem … but it *is* a link worth making.

CASE REPORT
A 38 year old woman had a past history of seven, possibly eight miscarriages. She complained of skin irritation, and, later, ulceration in the skin of the legs. Conventional treatment (support stockings etc.) was unsuccessful. Investigations turned up a highly positive aPL. For nearly 48 months no specific treatment was given and the ulcers worsened. After a case conference, it was decided to start Warfarin. The ulcers healed and have remained healed. As this stage, the anticoagulation has been continued, largely at the patient's request.

The Blood

The blood abnormality described in our 1983 papers was low platelets ("thrombocytopenia"). Although this is a relatively uncommon event, it *is* important – and another feature which distinguishes Hughes' syndrome from other clotting disorders.

At first sight, the presence of a low platelet count seems odd. Low platelets are associated with *bleeding*, not clotting. And yet in this syndrome the two can go together.

Figure 9.2 lists the normal and abnormal platelet ranges. As can be seen in this rather over-simplified scale, a platelet count of around 100 thousand, whilst technically low, is not a treatment problem.

Many patients with APS run platelet counts of around 100,000. Occasionally, however, the platelet count can drop and a real danger of bleeding, rather than clotting occurs.

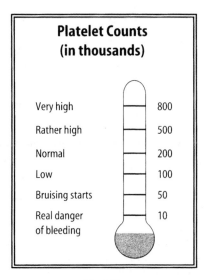

**Platelet Counts
(in thousands)**

Very high	800
Rather high	500
Normal	200
Low	100
Bruising starts	50
Real danger of bleeding	10

Fig. 9.2

CASE REPORT

A 33 year old teacher had previously had two episodes of leg thrombosis and investigations had shown a positive aPL. He was treated at first with Warfarin, but subsequently with long term low dose aspirin (75mgs daily). Following a school cricket match, he noticed more-than-expected bruising on his legs. He then complained of excessive gum bleeding. Investigations showed a platelet count of 4,000. He was treated for a period of 3 months with steroids (Prednisolone) and the platelet count returned to normal. There has been no subsequent episode of low platelets.

Oddly enough, there seem to be a group of aPL-positive individuals whose sole medical problem is with low platelet counts and (at least so far) with no clotting problems. Where these patients have a different mechanism or different form of the disease is unclear at present.

I will come back to the research and mechanisms of the illness later. It is worth pointing out that the platelet – an essential clotting component of blood, is basically a 2-skin envelope – each skin consisting of phospholipid. As in magnetic fields, there are "positive" charged phospholipids and "negative" charged. Any alteration of the status-quo can result in platelet changes – and either bleeding or clotting.

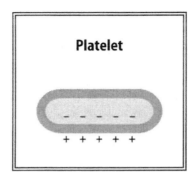

Fig. 9.3

Another surface of the blood which may be attacked, is the membrane of the red blood cell. Damage to the red cell membrane results in rupture of the cell, and to anaemia – so called "**haemolytic anaemia**". This form of "auto-immune" anaemia is a well recognised, though relatively rare form of the APS.

10 The "Catastrophic" Antiphospholipid Syndrome

This is the most feared complication of Hughes' syndrome. Fortunately, it is extremely rare – but when it occurs it is an "all stops out" medical emergency.

The most commonly cited scenario is in an individual with aPL who appears to be well – often on no treatment – who suddenly starts to develop widespread clots. The clots involve any or all of the vital organs – the lungs, the liver, the adrenals, the brain.

The patient becomes extremely ill and invariably requires intensive care treatment.

The triggering factor(s) for this "gear-change" is unknown, though in a number of patients an infection such as a virus, sore throat or chest infection seems to start the process. Another, rare, cause is the stopping of anticoagulant treatment in a known aPL patient.

CASE REPORT
A 35 year old woman, previously diagnosed as Hughes' syndrome with leg vein thrombosis, previous spontaneous abortions, livedo reticularis, and a number of small strokes, had been successfully treated with Warfarin (Coumadin) for 3 years and was doing very well. On Christmas Day she was involved in a car crash, suffered head injuries and was admitted unconscious to a neuro-surgical centre. Warfarin was stopped because of the danger of internal bleeding. After an initial improvement, she again started to become more drowsy and short of breath. A heart murmur was noted, and her liver function tests became abnormal. Her condition deteriorated rapidly, with lung and liver failure and wors-

ening heart valve function. In collaboration with our unit, it was decided to re-start anticoagulation. There was a clear and marked improvement. Two years later she underwent corrective valve surgery. The patient remains well 9 years after the Christmas emergency, and on life-long anticoagulants.

Because the catastrophic syndrome is so rare, there are few reports of successful treatment. Obviously, careful anticoagulation treatment is essential, as well as specialised intensive care management. Some studies have suggested that "blood-cleansing" (plasma exchange) might help by reducing the level of disease-producing antibodies. This makes good sense, but hard evidence for the success of this treatment is still lacking.

11 Pregnancy and Fetal Loss

For the purpose of clinical definition, pregnancy is divided into 2 halves, each of 20 weeks. Any pregnancy loss before 20 weeks is classified as abortion and after 20 weeks, when the fetus is well-formed, as fetal loss.

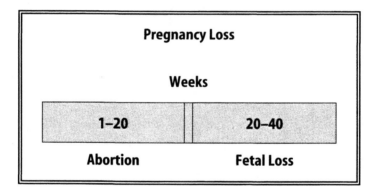

Pregnancy Loss

Weeks

1–20	20–40
Abortion	**Fetal Loss**

Fig. 11.1

One of the gains from the recognition of Hughes' syndrome is that it is a significant cause of spontaneous abortion and of fetal death. And it is a treatable cause.

The simple (possibly simplistic) theory as to the cause is that the "sticky blood" is unable to traverse the smallest blood vessels in the placenta. The placenta withers and the embryo/fetus fails to thrive and is aborted. This theory is supported by the finding of small, clotted placenta in many cases. However, in others, the placenta appears normal and perhaps other explanations may apply in these cases.

Secondly, spontaneous abortion is recognised as a relatively common "normal" event. In the majority, the reasons are unknown – possibly a significant number are due to nature's way of dealing with badly formed embryos. Nevertheless, the APS is a very treatable cause of recurrent pregnancy loss, often by as simple a medicine as one "junior" aspirin a day.

CASE REPORT

A 39 year old woman had suffered 11 spontaneous miscarriages. Following a clinical meeting on APS in 1982, her physician in Scotland sent blood to us for aPL and she was positive. She was treated with 75mgs aspirin daily and completed a successful pregnancy (followed by a second 1 year later).

This patient – a woman whose courage and determination was finally rewarded, used to travel down to London for her check-ups on the overnight train – a 20 hour round trip!

Fetal loss (loss of pregnancy after 20 weeks) is on the other hand, very rare. A woman with *recurrent* fetal loss *must* be checked for Hughes' syndrome, as this is an important and again preventable cause. Sadly, the disaster of fetal loss can occur late into the pregnancy – indeed one of the reasons for the huge improvement in pregnancy outcome in APS is the obstetric management of late pregnancy loss.

One of the advances in management has come with the use of Doppler monitor to screen blood flow to the fetus. This sensitive measure gives a clear indication of whether the pulse wave of blood to the fetus is healthy. One of the early warning signs of a failing, or clotting, circulation to the fetus is a falling off of the pulse wave.

The final and critical stage to the fetus is a reversal of blood flow. At this stage, emergency caesarean section is required. Many critical aPL pregnancies have been saved at this late stage because of Doppler information.

At the other end of the pregnancy – in the first weeks – early embryo loss can also occur. Clearly, recurrent early embryo loss can be misdiagnosed as "primary" infertility. The contribution of aPL to the list of causes of infertility is still very uncertain, but some I.V.F. clinics are taking note of the role of "sticky blood" being a contributing factor in some cases.

In summary, two very positive points should be emphasised. There is no lasting danger to the baby. For example, the blood vessels of the newborn baby are fine, and unaffected by the syndrome. Secondly, APS has proved an enormous success for literally thousands of mothers. In most centres, the success rate for APS pregnancies has risen from under 20% to a remarkable 75%.

Testing for antiphospholipid antibodies is becoming routine in obstetric clinics around the world. Whereas once it was a blood test thought only to be required in a patient who had had two or more pregnancies losses, nowadays it is becoming more and more a "routine" screening test. There is much to be said for this. For the relatively small costs involved, many pregnancies could be saved, often with as safe a medicine as junior aspirin.

12 Hughes' Syndrome and Lupus

Lupus is a major disease of the immune system, in which a wide variety of antibodies are produced. It is being increasingly recognised throughout the world, and in some countries in the Far East and in the Caribbean, it has overtaken rheumatoid arthritis in prevalence.

It affects females more than males (9 : 1) and at a relatively young age (15–50).

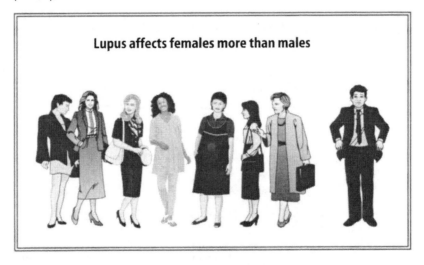

Lupus affects females more than males

Fig. 12.1

The abnormalities of the immune system can affect any and every organ in the body, including the joints, the skin (skin rashes), the kidneys, the brain and the blood vessels. Thrombosis can be a complication of the disease, and, in pregnancy, there is a slightly increased risk of miscarriage.

41

(There are a number of patients' books on lupus, including "Lupus – the facts" (Oxford University Press).

Whilst studying aspects of lupus in the 1970's, we found that one group of antibodies (antiphospholipid antibodies – aPL) were strongly associated with thrombosis in lupus. Indeed, the association was so strong that the antibodies were felt to clearly define a subgroup of lupus patients with a special disease pattern. For example, lupus pregnancies without aPL did *not* have a higher incidence of miscarriage.

We went on to show that aPL were also found in patients *without* lupus – a syndrome we named the primary antiphospholipid syndrome ("Primary APS"). What are the relationships between the two conditions? The answer is shown in simplified form in Figure 12.2 – a so-called Venn diagram.

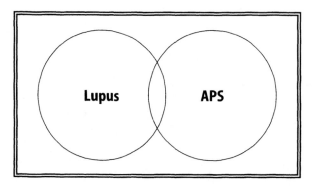

Fig. 12.2

There is overlap. Depending, obviously, on the sensitivity of the tests, a proportion of lupus patients (perhaps 20%) have aPL and features of the antiphospholipid syndrome.

This leaves on either side, two large groups, one with "classical" lupus, and the other with "primary APS" (i.e., no evidence of lupus).

I have shown the 2 groups to be similar size, though, as yet, no one is sure of the relative frequencies of the 2 diseases. However, we do have a partial answer to the question asked by many patients with Hughes' syndrome – "Will I go on to develop lupus?". The answer in general is "no".

We have been following a large number of APS patients now for up to 20 years, and it is notably that transition to lupus is *rare* – very rare. As distinct from lupus, some Hughes' syndrome patients do have other autoimmune disorders. The two most commonly associated disorders are thyroid problems, often mild, and a disorder called Sjogren's syndrome.

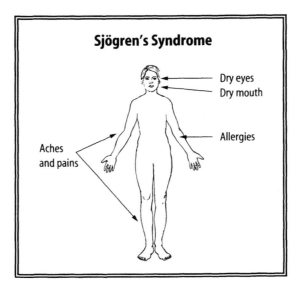

Fig. 12.3

This is a disorder characterised by dryness and irritation of the eyes and dryness of the mouth, together with a tendency to aches and pains. Sjogren's is often so mild that it passes undiagnosed.

13 Treatment

There are two logical approaches to treatment – either to suppress the antibodies (aPL) which cause the trouble, or to go for the end result and treat the clotting tendency itself – with some form of anticoagulant. In practice it is only the second form of treatment which has proved effective, i.e., treatment with aspirin, warfarin (coumadin) or heparin. These will be discussed first.

Aspirin

"Low dose" aspirin (75 – 100mgs daily) has long been found to be effective in reducing platelet stickiness. It is now used throughout the world on a daily basis by people concerned about clotting problems – for example, in those who have had previous heart attacks.

Interestingly, 1999 marked the 100th anniversary of aspirin and its development by Bayer; and it is fitting that this "new" syndrome – APS – is now being added to the potential uses of the drug.

There is no doubt that aspirin is effective. For example, in pregnancy, the miscarriage rate has fallen dramatically – more, in our own experience, due to aspirin than to any other single factor.

Obviously, for those with less severe problems, aspirin 75mgs daily (80 or 100mgs in some countries) is the safest form of prophylaxis against further problems. It may also be shown one day that aspirin is an effective preventor of clots in otherwise asymptomatic aPL positive individuals.

Some of the other features, for example, headaches, are sometimes helped by a daily low dose aspirin regime.

CASE REPORT

A 27 year old woman with mild lupus was troubled with frequent migraine-like headaches. She had not had any previous thrombosis and her brain scan was normal. She was aPL positive. A course of 75mgs aspirin daily was started on a trial-and-error basis, with a marked decrease in frequency of the headaches.

The most common side-effect of aspirin is indigestion, though this tiny dose rarely causes problems. A rare, though potentially serious problem is aspirin allergy (including asthma) and here aspirin may have to be substituted by an alternative anti-platelet drug such as dipyrimidole.

For more major problems, including recent vein and artery thrombosis or stroke, aspirin alone is insufficient and anticoagulation with heparin or warfarin is needed.

Warfarin

This drug, also known as coumadin, is important in the treatment of Hughes' syndrome, and is very effective.

It has often had something of a bad press – "rat poison", etc. – but provided the blood tests are carefully monitored, patients generally take the medicine for years (many for life) without problems.

Warfarin is an anticoagulant. It results in thinning of the blood. The dose is found by a process of trial and error, the aim being to keep the blood "twice as thin" or "three times as thin" as normal.

The measurement used is the "INR" (internationally normalised ratio) which compares the patients blood to normal blood. Rather like half cream milk (INR 2) or one third cream milk (INR 3). Thus, the higher the ratio, the thinner the blood.

Most patients with APS keep an INR of between 2 to 3 – in some patients it needs to be thinner still – 3.5 to 4. The control is monitored using anti-coagulant "cards" or "diaries" giving dosage and INR results.

The only major side-effect of warfarin is bleeding – almost always when the anticoagulant control has gone wrong. It is important to remember that some foods, alcohol and especially drugs (e.g., antibiotics) interfere with warfarin dosage.

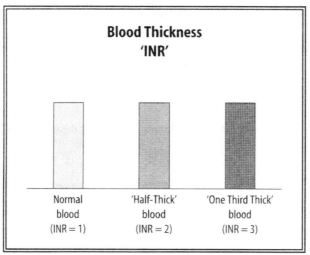

Fig. 13.1

As many of the case reports in this book testify, getting the warfarin dosage right can result in marked clinical benefit. Once adequate anti-coagulant control is achieved, the patient with APS can hopefully return to a normal existence.

Heparin

This drug acts differently from warfarin, and has two major limitations – firstly, it must be given by injection. Secondly, if given over a prolonged period of time, it can cause bone softening (osteoporosis). Heparin is used in three main situations. Firstly, it is used in the immediate aftermath of thrombosis, in view of its rapid action. Secondly, it is used around the time of surgery (or obstetric delivery) as its action can be switched on and off more quickly than warfarin. Thirdly, it is used where anticoagulation is required in pregnancy. Warfarin is toxic to the developing fetus, and it therefore not used in pregnancy – at least not in the first half of pregnancy.

Over the past 14 years, there has been a change in prescribing patterns with heparin. Now "low molecular weight" heparin is commercially available and, certainly in our clinics, has replaced the older form. These preparations, which include calcium heparin (Calciparine), enoxaparin (Clexane), dalteparin (Fragmin) and tinzaparin (Innohep), have a number of advantages. They can easily be self-administered by patients using pre-packed small needle syringes (similar to diabetic insulin syringes). They have a more "even" spread of action and can be given once or twice daily. In pregnancy, they do not cross the placenta, and thus, do not endanger the fetus.

Other Drugs

Intravenous Immunoglobulin (IVIG)

This consists of an intravenous preparation of protein (globulin) pooled from a large number of donors. It is extremely expensive, and its action is short-lived. Some years ago, it was found to help in some cases of thrombocytopenia (low platelets) and has since been used in a variety of auto-immune diseases with mixed success. Despite its apparent limitations, it has a good safety record, and is being tried in some patients with Hughes' syndrome, particularly those with low platelet counts.

Immunosuppressives

These drugs (most commonly azathioprine and methotrexate) are widely used in auto-immune diseases such as lupus and rheumatoid arthritis. They have proved disappointing in patients with primary APS. So also has plasma exchange – an attractive idea for removing antibodies, but with no convincing published success – as yet.

Antimalarials

Hydroxychloroquine (Plaquenil) is an extremely useful drug in lupus and Sjogren's syndrome. It is particularly effective in helping skin rashes, fatigue, and aches and pains. One of the additional actions of Plaquenil is as a (mild) anti-clotting agent – rather like junior aspirin. Thus, in lupus patients with aPL it might well have extra, hidden, benefits.

Treatment in Pregnancy

One thing is certain. Treatment of APS pregnancy has been one of the most successful aspects of the whole story. Women who had had 5, 10 even 12 or 15 miscarriages, are now having successful pregnancies. The success rate in pregnancy has risen from under 20% to over 70%.

This improvement is almost certainly due to a combination of medical and obstetric factors. In medicine, the main treatment decisions lie between the use of aspirin alone or aspirin plus heparin. For those women with recurrent miscarriages but with no previous thrombosis, our approach is to use aspirin 75mgs daily. For those with previous thrombosis, we use aspirin together with heparin. This is not the place to go into dosage regimes. However, there are now extensive trials going on to compare aspirin alone without heparin, or combined aspirin and heparin.

For patients with previous thrombosis on warfarin who wish to plan a pregnancy, our advice is to continue the warfarin until the pregnancy test becomes positive, then immediately to change to heparin.

General Treatment

There are three groups of individuals – those with antibodies but with no thrombosis, those with thrombosis of the veins, and the most serious group, those with strokes and artery clots. Most doctors recommend low dose daily aspirin for "asymptomatic" aPL positive individuals. However, some of the studies mentioned earlier suggest that some go on to develop clots *despite* aspirin. Our research unit is currently conducting a prospective, European wide study comparing the use of aspirin with very low dose Warfarin in this group. The study will take 5 years, but we hope that it will answer some important questions. At the present time, my best advice is to use daily aspirin, 75mgs daily.

For an individual with deep vein thrombosis (DVT), the conventional treatment is 6 months' warfarin – with "dilution of blood to half (an INR of 2). However, if aPL are present, clinical experience suggests the chances of re-thrombosing are higher, and it is conventional now to continue treatment for at least a year, and with a INR nearer 2.5

For those with artery thrombosis, including strokes, we believe that lifelong anticoagulants are probably needed. In a large study looking back at our patients, we found that in this group of patients, the only clearly effective treatment was strong anticoagulation – with an INR of 3 or more. Clearly, the risk of bleeding increases with this form of treatment – but this risk must be balanced against the far greater risk of further strokes.

Finally, there are very occasional patients in whom the combination of Warfarin and junior aspirin is helpful.

CASE REPORT

A 42 year old woman with Hughes' syndrome and recurrent severe headaches and a number of small strokes improved on Warfarin. However, after several months' treatment, and despite an INR kept stable between 3 and 3.5, the headaches returned. Aspirin 75mgs daily was added, with disappearance of the headaches. A number of attempts to stop the aspirin resulted in a return of the headaches.

Even in the short time that we have known about the syndrome, lessons have been learned. Firstly, do not under estimate the significance of a positive test in the present of suggestive clinical features. Treatment here is worthwhile.

Secondly, tests are not always high in all patients – in a considerable number of our patients the antibody levels gradually subside. Perhaps these individuals can finally stop medication.

Thirdly, careful treatment really is very worthwhile. A good number of my "early" patients seen 20 years ago, at that time with serious medical complications, such as stroke, liver disease and leg ulcers, are now living a full and normal life.

14 The Outlook

This is difficult to predict, especially as it is less than 20 years since the syndrome was first described. Clinically, the clinical spectrum is huge, varying from no symptoms ("asymptomatic carriers of aPL"), to multiple strokes.

The more I see of the syndrome, the more seriously I take it. Obviously, it is quite possible in a referral centre such as mine to see the worst patients and get a slanted view. But the disaster of a major thrombosis which *could* have been prevented does argue strongly for some sort of treatment, even in the mildest cases.

There have been some studies on prognosis, though as yet these studies have a number of limitations. One study from our unit carried out a 10 year look-back at patients seen in 1986 – "the class of 86". In general, this group of patients, seen by us at that time, were lupus patients or women with recurrent miscarriage found to have aPL. Most of the patients had been followed up in our clinic over the decade. The results were striking. Just over *one half* of the patients developed a thrombosis of one sort or another – strong support for the argument that aPL positive individuals should be closely monitored.

The major advance as far as Hughes' syndrome is concerned is *diagnosis*. It is becoming abundantly clear that once adequate treatment is started, the disease can often be stopped in its tracks. This begs the question of what *is* the most appropriate treatment? And for how long?

The feeling of most doctors treating APS patients is where there has been a *major* thrombosis, especially thrombosis of an artery or a stroke, anticoagulation should be life-long. For those with a less severe vein thrombosis, the period of anticoagulation with Warfarin can be much shorter, e.g., 6 months to a year.

For those with positive tests and *no* thrombosis, (and this group includes those diagnosed following miscarriage), the long-term management is less certain. Some advocate no treatment, others long-term aspirin. Hopefully, the number of prospective trials now in progress may provide some answers to these questions.

15 What Blood Tests Do We Use?

In theory there should be one simple blood test. In practice, there are two. These are (1) the *anticardiolipin* test, and (2) the *"lupus anticoagulant"*.

A third test – once used to test for syphylis, the so-called VDRL or WR – is also found positive in a small percentage of patients.

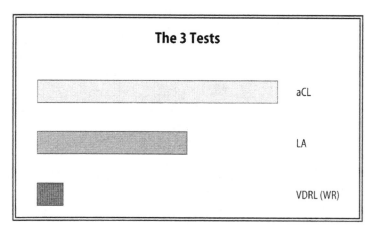

Fig. 15.1

Although the tests measure broadly the same thing, there are a small number (perhaps 10%) where one or other test is negative. In other words, one test alone could miss the diagnosis.

Anticardiolipin Antibodies

This is a simple, very reproducible test which costs a few dollars, and is performed in most major centres throughout the world. Many labs use semi-standardised "kits" on a "mass production" basis.

A drop of blood serum is placed on a glass plate containing protein and phospholipid (there are a variety of phospholipids, but "cardiolipin" – partly because of its easy availability – is used). A positive test is read out on a standard photometry ("ELISA") meter.

Conventionally, "low" positive readings are between 0 and 15 (IgG) units, "medium" between 15 and 50 units, and "high" over 50 units. For those involved in trials and research, two positive readings, 6 months apart are needed. Positive readings are rarely seen in other conditions – hence the test is fairly specific.

Lupus Anticoagulant

The APS was first fully described in lupus patients (see Chapter 1). All large series of lupus patients had included thrombosis, recurrent abortion, stroke – and so on – in their reported clinical features.

One test, described half a century ago, was the confusingly named "lupus anticoagulant". This is now known to be an antibody – in fact, one of the family of aPL, which interferes with clotting. Its name is *wrong*. We had all hoped that this complicated and wrongly-named test would simply go away, and be replaced by newer, simpler tests. Not quite yet, unfortunately.

More significantly, a test used in the old days for syphilis – the "Wasserman" reaction – basically a test for aPL, was found to give embarrassing "false positive" tests in some lupus patients. We now know that the "false positive" syphilis test once seen in lupus patients was probably what we now recognise as the aPL which we test today.

Other Tests

As always, the science gets more complicated rather than easier. In 1990, three groups of researchers found that the antibodies bound not to phospholipids alone, but to proteins, which in turn bound to phospholipids! Some of these proteins – "Beta-2 glycoprotein 1" and "prothrombin" are being used in some assays, but for the most part, these tests are experimental and not used in routine practice.

For the practitioner investigating a diagnosis of Hughes' syndrome, the main tests are the *anticardiolipin antibody* and, to a lesser extent, the *lupus anticoagulant.*

I know from my own experience, and from that of my colleagues, that these 2 tests are available in most major clinics throughout the world.

16 Research

There is a huge international research effort underway into the mechanisms and treatment of Hughes' syndrome. One of the bonuses of working in this disease has been the degree of collaboration world-wide. Our own unit for example, has published collaborative studies with colleagues in Japan, Spain, Italy, Brazil, Mexico, Israel, Holland, America and France. The regular international meetings are truly constructive, and the publications in international journals such as "LUPUS" reflect the teamwork and the huge expansion in knowledge of this subject.

Some of the main areas of research are listed here.

Geography

There are reports and series published from all over the world. However, the study of "epidemiology" or geography of a disease sometimes turns up differences which provide clues to the causes of a disease. For example, the "stiff back" syndrome called spondylitis has long been known to be common in northern parts of Europe and America, and very rare in black Africa. It subsequently become known that this genetic disease was strongly associated with a certain blood group (HLA B27) and that the geography of this blood group mirrored the geographic pattern of the disease.

In Hughes' syndrome there are some suggestions of geographic and ethnic differences, but at present these are few and far between. One interesting study from Professor Malawiya in Kuwait suggested that the disease was more prevalent in the Arabic community than in the Indian community there.

A number of colleagues in the USA and in the Caribbean have suggested that the disease might be less common in blacks than whites – an interesting difference from lupus, if this observation proves to be true.

Genetics

"My mother suffered from migraines and my sister also had a number of miscarriages". From the first descriptions of the syndrome in 1983, there has been no doubt that evidence of a possible genetic tendency exists in some families. The tendency is not strong – the majority of our patients do not give a clear history of positive family histories. Nevertheless, as with other "autoimmune diseases", all of which are known to have a genetic basis, a number of studies point to a similar background in APS. Dozens of collaborative studies are currently in progress in centres all over the world, and it is likely that in the not-too-distant future, the genetic "fingerprint" predisposing to APS will be better known.

The Immune System

The common thread linking patients with Hughes' syndrome is the presence of antibodies which react to phospholipid-proteins. Antibodies are proteins circulating in the blood, which normally have the task of defending against foreign "invaders" such as viruses and bacteria.

In healthy people, following an infection, antibodies are produced for a period of time sufficient to either neutralise or, in other ways, to destroy the infection. When the danger is over, the immune system stops producing the antibodies, which then slowly disappear from the circulation.

In the so-called "auto-immune" diseases such as lupus, the antibody production continues relentlessly – and apparently aimlessly. The Sorcerer's apprentice.

The fundamental cause of this "over-revving" of the engine is unclear. Figure 16.1 shows our conventional concept of the antibody which seems to attach to a complicated mixture of protein and phospholipid.

Why the Clotting?

There are a number of theories – possibly all playing a part. One attractive theory is that the antibodies influence the blood platelets. Platelets essentially consist of two membranes ("sausage skins") made largely of phospholipids. Alterations of these membranes could theoretically lead to platelet stickiness and clotting.

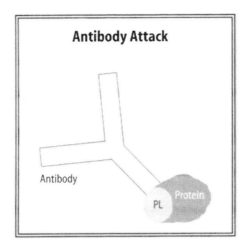

Fig. 16.1

Another "membrane" is the inside lining of the blood vessels – the so-called endothelium. A number of studies have already shown that aPL can alter endothelial cell membranes. Any alteration of the inside lining of the blood vessel makes it more prone to develop thrombosis.

A third, and equally possible explanation, is that the antibodies affect the actual clotting proteins of the blood.

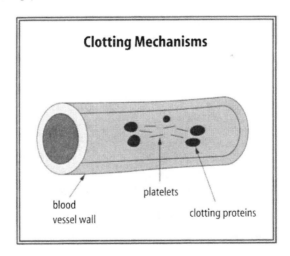

Fig. 16.2

However, the biggest question remains unsolved – why don't patients with the antibodies clot *all* the time? One favoured explanation is the "two hit" phenomenon. As well as the antibodies, a second (or third) risk factor is required. One such risk factor is infection, which itself is known to affect some of the mechanisms mentioned above and which, in some individuals, may be the trigger which sets off the thrombosis.

Clinical Studies

The clinical impact of the syndrome is huge. In obstetrics, it is a (treatable) cause of 20%, or even more, of recurrent miscarriages. It is a (treatable) cause of up to 1 in 5 strokes in younger individuals. It also impinges on so many other conditions. For example, it may be a "cause" of multiple sclerosis – of migraine – of memory loss – of oral contraceptive induced thrombosis – of infertility – of leg ulcers – of raised blood pressure : all with an identifiable and preventable cause.

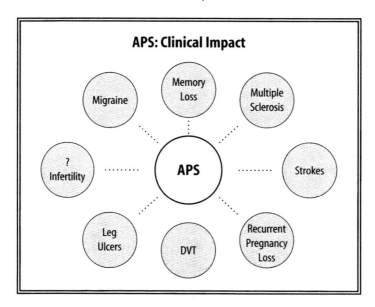

Fig. 16.3

Clinicians looking after these conditions are recognising that a simple blood screening test – antiphospholipid antibodies – may point some – possibly many – of their patients towards more effective treatment.

One of the clinical developments during the past ten years is the recognition that the syndrome may provide clues to the world-wide problem of artery disease – atheroma. The interactions of these antibodies with lipids, blood vessels and accelerated arterial disease is one of the key areas in research in APS.

Treatment

Put bluntly, the treatment options – warfarin (coumadin), heparin or aspirin – sound limited. They are, but the careful and precise use of these treatments has changed life for the better in so many patients.

Yes, it would be nice if we could be more "fundamental" in our treatment, and get rid of the offending antibodies. This is not easy with present treatments, but research is going on to find newer "selective" ways of either removing antibodies (by "selective plasmapheresis" or "selective immunosuppression") – by raising antidotes to the specific problem antibodies – suppressing these antibodies alone and not "poisoning" the whole bone marrow.

There are other approaches. Could diet help? Certainly any disease of blood vessels where "lipids" are involved in worthy of dietary study. Although no major studies are yet published, a number of groups are working in this area. Do vitamins help? The term "oxidised" is now used a lot and there is some evidence that certain foods and drugs (vitamin E, for example) which have "anti-oxidant" properties could well stave off artery disease.

So at present, it is mainly back to diagnosis and, in turn, the prevention of the widespread consequences of "sticky blood". The finding of antiphospholipid antibodies is already proving to be on of the most clinically significant tests in the practice of medicine.

17 Background

Most of our early work in describing the antiphospholipid syndrome (APS) came from studies of a disease called **Lupus**. Lupus is a disease in which the immune system goes into "over-drive" and produces a huge variety of excess antibodies. Lupus is a common and important disease, mainly affecting young women, and seen in almost every country in the world. Once thought rare, it is now recognised as a major disease, commoner than, for example, multiple sclerosis or leukaemia, and in some countries, overtaking rheumatoid arthritis in prevalence.

For many years scientists have researched on the reaction of certain antibodies on brain. In 1975 I was invited to set up a rheumatology clinic in the University of the West Indies with my research fellow, Dr Wendel Wilson. We saw an enormous number of lupus patients there : lupus in all its forms. One disease which interested us was a form of tropical paralysis called Jamaican neuropathy. This disastrous spinal paralysis, now known to be due to a virus, showed some interesting parallels to lupus, with anti-nuclear antibodies, and, more interestingly, with antibodies directed against phospholipids – molecules important in the structure and composition of the nervous system. We hypothesised that antiphospholipid antibodies might interfere with *brain* tissue and might directly result in disease.

We carried out these studies, both in Jamaican neuropathy and then in our lupus patients, first at Hammersmith Hospital, and subsequently in St Thomas' Hospital in London.

As so often happens, we found something rather different from our original focus on brain tissue. We found that these antibodies were strongly – *very* strongly – associated with a tendency to thromboses, including placental thrombosis and miscarriage. We presented these findings in a number of meetings in the late '70's and early 80's, and in the years 1983, 1984 and 1985 published a number of papers detailing the full breadth of the syndrome, including the important observation that *arteries* as well as veins could clot.

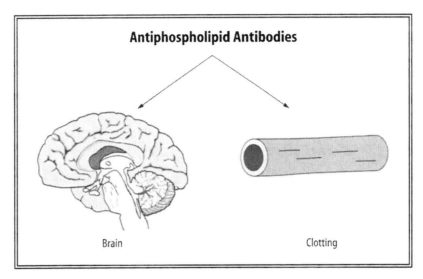

Fig. 17.1

We recognised early on that the syndrome could exist in the *absence* of lupus. This "primary" syndrome, which we first named the "anticardiolipin syndrome" (after the cardiolipin test which we used) and subsequently re-named "primary antiphospholipid syndrome" is an important and common condition, seen in clinics in all branches of medicine, from obstetrics to neurology. In my opinion (and only time will tell) the syndrome will come to be recognised as more common than lupus, and a major – and largely preventable – disease world-wide.

Thirdly, largely due to the efforts of three of my pupils and collaborators, Dr Nigel Harris, Dr Aziz Gharavi and Dr Munther Khamashta, we set up precise assays for antibody testing, collaborative workshops, and, in 1984 and 1986, the first 2 International Conferences – conferences which now, every 2 years, attract research workers from all over the world and result in important scientific publications (see literature list).

I would like to mention, in particular, 3 of these conferences. In Italy in 1990 in the conference organised by Dr Angela Tincani and her colleagues, a major breakthrough come in the understanding of the clotting mechanism – the discovery of the so called "co-factor".

In the 1995 Louvain meeting, organised by Drs Arnout and Vermylen, a number of colleagues proposed re-naming the syndrome "Hughes' Syndrome". I am grateful to these colleagues for this honour.

In the 1998 conference, organised by Professor T Koike in Sapporo, Japan, an important set of international criteria were drawn up, to help standardise the collaborative work going on in this syndrome.

18 Further Reading and Websites

1. Textbook

HUGHES' SYNDROME – Antiphospholipid Syndrome.
M A Khamashta, Editor. Springer-Verlag, London 2000

2. Conference Report

Proceedings of the 8th International Antiphospholipid Conference (Sapporo, Japan), Koike T, Editor
LUPUS 1998, Vol 7, Suppl. 2
Papers and abstracts from the 9th International Antiphospholipid Conference (Tours, France) Boffa M-C and Piette J-C Editors.
Journal of Autoimmunity 2000, Vol. 15, No. 2

3. References

Hughes' Syndrome: The Antiphospholipid Syndrome. A historical view.
Reprinted with permission from LUPUS 1998, 7 suppl 2, S1 – S4
Speculations on APS in the coming Millennium.
Reprinted with permission from Journal of Autoimmunity 2000 Vol. 15 (No. 2) pp 269–271

4. Websites

www.lupus.org.uk
www.hughes-syndrome.org
> (This website provides updated information on research and treatment, a question and answer section and details of patient support group membership).